"I'm looking for a weight management program I can do in my home when it is most convenient for me." "My hectic lifestyle does not leave much time for me to go to the fitness center to work out." If that sounds familiar to you, this book is for you. In this book, you will find a weight management program designed for beginners that can be achieved at home when it is most convenient for you. All you need is the desire to lose weight and keep it off.

About the Author

Stephen is the twelfth child of Elder John and Annie Wright. He was born in Quincy, Florida and graduated from James A. Shanks High School. He received a B.S. degree from the University of South Alabama and an M.A. degree from Webster University. Desiring to see the world and experience new cultures, he joined the Air Force and faithfully served for twenty-four years. The experiences he learned abroad fueled his enthusiasm to write. Stephen is married to the former Diane Hughes of Prichard, Alabama.

Sauveur

What if everything you have learned about politics was a lie? Finley Michaelson accidentally uncovered a conspiracy protected by an oath of secrecy dating back to the 1700s that mandated all U.S. Presidents be descendants of a royal bloodline. The conspiracy was led by a group called Sauveur who was willing to die to protect the secret. Understanding it was their birthright to civilize those they considered as inferior, they deployed a relentless campaign to silence the minority races. For centuries, Sauveur's ultimate conspiracy of controlling the White House was never challenged until a Presidential election involving a minority candidate. In the wake of the largest conspiracy in American history, the existence of the most powerful organization in the world was threatened by a single post on social media.

***

Retribution: Some Friends Can't Be Trusted

Were you betrayed by a friend? After the suspicious death of her husband, Kuwanyauma was pursued by a secret organization with deadly intentions. Realizing some friends can't be trusted, Kuwanyauma dispensed her brand of justice...Retribution.

***

One Last Prayer

What will you do to prevent your best friend from being abused? As a child, Wanda witnessed her father repeatedly abuse her mother. She sought refuge in the church to ensure she wouldn't be involved in an abusive relationship. One Sunday, she met Abigail and they immediately became friends and eventually attended the same college. One frightful night, Abigail was attacked in her dorm room. Faced with the nightmares of her childhood, Wanda was forced to make a dreadful decision.

***

Zoey

Mrs. Lewis was a narcissist. As a child, she was told she was perfect and only accepted perfection. The granddaughter of wine producers in France and the daughter of a breeder of purebred American Alsatians, she was surrounded by wealth and perfection. A TV news anchorwoman and married to St. Louis' top Veterinarian, she was admired by millions. One Thanksgiving, her life was turned upside down after her daughter's four-minute seizure. Unable to accept imperfection, Mrs. Lewis struggled to accept her daughter's new lifestyle. A heartwarming story about a special bond between a girl and her dog with an inspiring ending.

***

Lose Weight At Home: A Beginner's Guide to Weight Loss

Have you tried to lose weight only to regain the weight you lost and more? Are you too busy to visit a fitness center due to the demands of your family? Do you constantly make excuses why you can't lose weight and keep it off? Are you looking for a weight management program you can complete at home at your convenience? If you answered "yes" to these questions, this book is for you.

***

The Carcian Chronicle

For more than a century after the foretelling of his birth, Guardians from planet Carci scoured planet Earth to locate The One, the Great Warrior. Born with an IQ of 180 to a barren mother, he achieved greatness at an early age. Aided by Guardians, not from his world, he fulfilled his destiny.

Unknown to him, fulfilling his destiny on planet Earth was only half of the prophecy. With all memories of planet Earth erased during rebirth, the Great Warrior, accompanied by his Protector, set out to fulfill the prophecy.

Angered by the destruction of his Protector and a total memory recall, he realized nothing was as it seemed. To accept his future, he had to come to grips with his past.

As foretold by the prophecy, a traitor conspired to rule the galaxy. Abducting humans from planet Earth and transforming them to Leets, programmable warriors with telepathic abilities, the traitor led his warriors into battle; a battle between Guardians and Leets.

Available at www.amazon.com, www.createspace.com, or through my website at
https://www.stephenmwrightbooks.com.

WHAT WOULD YOU ATTEMPT TO DO IF YOU KNEW YOU WOULDN'T FAIL?

That is a very compelling question. Normally, the reason we are hesitant to try something new is that we are afraid to fail. If we are afraid to fail, we are also afraid to try. Numerous failures preceded all major accomplishments. _Failure is always an option._ To think otherwise, you have already failed.

To my lovely wife for her absolute support.

Introduction

Before I get started, let me tell you a little about me. I am not a Physician or Dietician/Nutritionist. Even though I have a Bachelor's degree in Physical Education, I do not consider myself an Expert or a Fitness Guru. I am just like you; someone who wants to maintain their weight at the desired level and increase their quality of life.

Who is the targeted audience for this book? This book is for those that have finally decided they want to improve their quality of life through weight loss. It is for anyone who has tried over and over to lose weight only to regain the weight they lost and more. It is for those of you that are embarrassed by your current physical appearance. For those of you who have purchased every aerobic DVD and every piece of "lose weight fast" exercise equipment on the market and stored them in your closet or under your bed, this book is for you.

Last and most important, it is for those that have been creative in coming up with excuses why they don't exercise such as "I don't have time to go to the gym." Whether you are trying to lose five pounds or fifty pounds, this program may help you achieve your goal if you truly want to manage your weight.

What will you accomplish by reading this book? Reading this book, you will learn how to manage your weight over a lifetime by changing your lifestyle. You will receive instructions on a program you can complete at your pace (please consult a physician before starting this program) inside your home without the use of expensive equipment or electronic devices. _This book does not promise immediate weight loss. If you are expecting immediate weight loss, this book is not for you._

To Lose or Not to Lose. That's ALWAYS the Question

If you search the web, you will find numerous statistics on how many people are overweight or obese. Most of us don't have to search the web because we see firsthand the signs of improper weight management. Maybe it's a member of your family or a close friend. *Maybe it's you*. Statistics is useful, but the statistic you are probably concerned about the most is your statistic. Are you overweight or obese?

The answer to that question is critical if you want to manage your weight. You have to decide if you actually wish to lose weight. *You have to admit you have a problem in order to seek a solution for it*. If you are overweight, and you are happy being overweight, I applaud you. *Not everyone can maintain their ideal weight, but everyone deserves to be happy*. If you are not satisfied with your current weight, you need to do something about it. *You will not lose weight and keep it off if you don't think your weight is a problem.*

According to Merriam-Webster, the definition of overweight is "excessive or burdensome weight, " and the definition of obese is "having excessive body fat." The term "overweight" also refers to a person that is above their *"ideal"* weight. I know the question you are asking is "what is my ideal weight?"

Your ideal weight is what you should weigh based on your age, height, and sex. If you search the web, you will find many sites with calculators to help you decide your *ideal* weight. Words of caution: *the information you find may be very discouraging.* The focus of this book is not your ideal weight. This book discusses how to maintain your *desired* weight, the weight you *want* to achieve.

What you will not find in this book are charts telling you what your ideal weight is because if you are like me, you will never achieve that goal. Weight loss requires a realistic and honest approach. The first step to solving a problem is to admit a problem exists. *To lose weight, you have to admit you are overweight and want to make a change.* You have taken the first step because if you are reading this book, you have already decided you weigh more than you want to weigh.

Goal Setting

To begin the process of weight loss, you need to create goals. Goals help you keep track of your progress. You need to create long and short range goals. While on active duty in the Air Force, I learned how to create SMART goals. Let's discuss the SMART acronym.

S – Specific
M – Measurable
A – Achievable
R – Relevant
T – Time-bound

Specific: When you create your goals, you need to be specific about what you want to accomplish. "I want to lose weight" is not a good goal. "I will lose twenty-four pounds in twelve months" is a good goal and is considered as your "long range" goal. You stated what you would accomplish and set a time frame to accomplish it in. You can be more specific by setting a particular date. "I will lose twenty-four pounds before 5/7/2015."

Measurable: Your goals should be measurable. You have stated you will lose twenty-four pounds in twelve months but how to know if you are on track to achieve your goal? You have to include "short range" goals to measure your performance. "I will lose two pounds every month" is an excellent way to measure your performance to ensure you stay on track.

   Achievable: This is a problem area for most people when they are trying to lose weight. You need to make sure your goals are possible. Creating a goal to lose 100 pounds in three months is unrealistic and very unhealthy. Your goals should be what you are striving to accomplish, but they have to be achievable. When you set an unrealistic goal, you will lose your motivation to achieve it and eventually discontinue the program.

   Relevant: Your goals need to be relevant. "I will not eat red meat" is not an appropriate weight loss goal. While decreasing your intake of red meat may be a good start to healthier living, your goals should pertain to weight loss.

   Time-Bound: Your goals need to have a completion date. In the example above, I said "twenty-four months" or "5/7/2015" which is your target date to accomplish your goal.

   After setting a goal, should you change it? You should tailor your goals to fit your needs. If you set a goal and realize it is *unachievable*, adjust it as necessary. A word of caution: "DO NOT ADJUST GOALS BECAUSE YOU FAILED TO REACH YOUR SHORT RANGE GOAL." If you failed to achieve your short range goal, you should change your approach to achieving your goal instead of changing the goal.

Goal Attainment

You have set your goal, and now it is time to accomplish it. Losing weight and keeping it off is a lifetime process and requires a change in lifestyle. *Quick weight loss typically leads to rapid weight gain*. You need to lose weight over time while changing your lifestyle to allow your body the opportunity to adjust to the new you.

When you are ready to start this program, *weigh yourself*. It will be your initial weight. You need to weigh yourself on a regular basis. I suggest you create a log to keep track of your initial weight and all of your future weight-ins. It is normal for your weight to fluctuate a pound or two daily. If you weigh weekly, you should see a gradual progression towards your goal. *To be successful with any weight management program, you need to enjoy it and be true to yourself*. Now that you have recorded your initial weight let's discuss the process.

As I stated earlier, losing weight and keeping it off requires a lifestyle change. It is something you have to continue for the rest of your life. This program is not a diet plan so I won't discuss weight loss through dieting. If you want information on dieting, contact a Dietician. Remember, *it's not what you eat but instead, when you eat it and how much you eat*.

Change your eating habits: Your goal should be to eat your last meal of the day *two to three hours* before bedtime to allow your food time to digest. It's a very difficult but significant step in managing your weight. If you currently get up in the middle of the night to eat, your starting point will be to eliminate the late night meal. Eating slowly and not overeating are also necessary steps in losing weight. If you eat slowly, your brain will inform you when you have eaten enough before you over eat. *Just because you have food left on your plate doesn't mean you have to eat it!*

One way to change your eating habits is to decrease the time of your last meal by one hour gradually until you can eat your last meal two to three hours before going to bed. I know some of you are coming up with many excuses why you can't do this. I'm sure I have heard all of them. *"I work late, so I have to eat late"* or *"I have to eat while watching TV."* Some of you may say *"I eat when I am angry"* or *"I can't sleep unless I eat right before going to bed."*

To be successful at weight loss, you need to *STOP MAKING EXCUSES*. As long as you can justify your eating habits, you will continue to do it. We are talking about a lifestyle change. It's a very time-consuming step and is the most important step in maintaining your weight. If you start and fail, try, try, and try again. If you want to lose weight and keep it off, you need to admit you have a problem and *STOP MAKING EXCUSES.*

If you usually go to bed at 11 PM, your *goal* should be to eat your last meal no later than 8 PM. *Should you try to eat your last meal no later than 8 PM on your first day in this program?* "NO!" If you do, you will inevitably fail. If you generally eat before going to bed at 11 PM, begin by eating your last meal at 10 PM.

Initially, this will be difficult because you are trying to break a long term habit. If you attempt and fail, try again. Continue until your body adjusts to it. There is no time limit to accomplish this so take as long as it takes for you to feel comfortable eating your last meal at 10 PM. Continue to weigh yourself and record data on your chart. *Always celebrate your small wins.*

When your body adjusts to eating at 10 PM, reduce your time to 9 PM. Initially, this will be difficult because you are trying to break a long term habit. If you attempt and fail, try again. Continue until your body adjusts to it. There is no time limit to accomplish this so take as long as it takes for you to feel comfortable eating your last meal at 9 PM.

Continue to weigh yourself and record data on your chart. *Always celebrate your small wins.* When your body adjusts to eating at 9 PM, reduce your time to 8 PM. Continue to reduce your time until you reach your goal. *Remember, if a medical emergency arises, seek medical attention immediately.*

Adjusting when you eat and how much you eat will help you achieve your *goal.* Tracking your weight weekly or as determined on your chart will show your progress. Initially, you will see exciting results and then the pounds will become harder to lose. If you have not lost any weight for two to three weeks, or you are gaining weight, it is time to adjust your routine. To do this, you can add some exercises to your routine.

Exercise

(Consult your Physician before starting this exercise regimen. If there is a feeling of discomfort any time while exercising, discontinue immediately and seek medical attention).

Now that you have gained control of your eating habits let's add a few exercises to help you reach your desired weight. *You should tailor your activities to what you are physically capable of achieving.* Some people make the mistake of overworking themselves on their first day at the fitness center by attempting to do a workout they see someone else doing instead of the workout they are capable of achieving. Most of the time, they never come back after the first day. For this program, you don't have to leave your home. You have to dedicate yourself to losing weight and realize if you cheat, *you are only cheating yourself.* Let's discuss the first exercise.

Walking: You probably don't think walking is a good exercise, but it is. One-third of my physical activity involves walking. I complete a 30-minute walk on the treadmill four times per week. My wife and I occasionally walk the neighborhood to exercise. Before beginning a walking routine, you need to set a goal of how long you want to walk.

This objective is not how long you will walk today but how long you will walk before a specified date. For example "I will walk sixty minutes a day by 5/7/2015". It requires a lifestyle change so don't set a goal you won't be able to achieve for the rest of your life. After setting your goal set short range goals and start at a pace you can maintain. If you can walk only one minute per day, walk one minute. Walk one minute per day until you can walk two. Walk two minutes per day until you can walk three.

Walk from room to room and up and down stairs. Continue this approach until you reach your goal. Taking this approach, you will continue to exercise because you will never overwork yourself. Eventually, you will reach your goal. When you have mastered walking inside and feel you are ready to go outside, start walking outside.

Don't be embarrassed to walk outside because you think people are talking about you because you are overweight. *Trust me, they are, but that's not your concern.* You are exercising for you, not them. Let them deal with their *ignorance* while you improve your quality of life. You need to commit to losing weight. You know how you look and feel right now and have decided you want to make a lifestyle change. Never lose focus on your goal. *Celebrate the small wins.*

You have changed your eating habits and eating early enough for your food to digest before going to bed and walking a specified amount of time daily. Walking does not replace your eating habits. To achieve maximum results, you need to continue to eat your last meal of the day two to three hours before bedtime while maintaining your walking regimen.

Take a look at your chart from time to time to remember your initial weight. If you have been dedicated and honest, you should see excellent results and be very proud of your accomplishments. Now it's time to add a few more exercises you can complete at home to your routine.

Leg Raise from a Sitting Position: Find a comfortable chair to sit on. Do not use a chair with armrests for this exercise. Set a goal you want to attain. *Your goal is not how many you wish to complete today but how many you will be able to complete before a specified date*. While sitting with your arms resting comfortably next to you raise one leg until it is horizontal to the floor and hold it in that position for three seconds if possible.

If you can't hold for three seconds, lower when necessary. When you lower your leg, raise the other leg until it is horizontal to the floor and hold it in that position for three seconds if possible. If you only complete one per leg today, that's okay.

Continue to increase the number of raises and the amount of time you can hold your leg in a raised position until you reach your goal. Your legs will be painful because you are working muscles that you don't typically work. As you continue, the pain should decrease. If a medical emergency arises while completing this exercise, discontinue and seek medical attention immediately.

Forward Arm Raise from a Sitting Position: Find a comfortable chair to sit on. Do not use a chair with armrests for this exercise. Set a goal you want to attain. *Your goal is not how many you wish to complete today but how many you will be able to complete before a specified date.* With your arms resting comfortably next to you, fully extend and raise one arm in front of you until it is horizontal to the floor and hold for three seconds if possible.

If you can't hold for three seconds, lower it when necessary. When you lower your arm, fully extend and raise the other arm in front of you until it is horizontal to the floor and hold it for three seconds if possible. If you can complete only one per arm today, that's okay.

Continue to increase the number of raises and the amount of time you can hold your arm in the raised position until you reach your goal. Your arms and shoulders will be painful because you are working muscles that you don't typically work. As you continue, the pain should decrease. If a medical emergency arises while completing this exercise, discontinue and seek medical attention immediately.

Lateral Arm Raise from a Sitting Position: Find a comfortable chair to sit on. Do not use a chair with armrests for this exercise. Set a goal you want to attain. *Your goal is not how many you wish to complete today but how many you will be able to complete before a specified date.* With your arms resting comfortably next to you, fully extend and raise one arm to the side until it is horizontal to the floor and hold for three seconds if possible.

If you can't hold for three seconds, lower it when necessary. When you lower your arm, fully extend and raise the other arm to the side until it is horizontal to the floor and hold it for three seconds if possible. If you only complete one per arm today, that's ok.

Continue to increase your number of raises and the amount of time you can hold your arm in the raised position until you reach your goal. Your arms and shoulders will be painful because you are working muscles that you don't typically work. As you continue, the pain should decrease. If a medical emergency arises while completing this exercise, discontinue and seek medical attention immediately.

Crunches from a Sitting Position: Find a comfortable chair to sit on. Set a goal you want to attain. *Your goal is not how many you wish to complete today but how many you will be able to complete before a specified date*. While sitting, exhale. While exhaling, tighten your abdomen muscles as much as possible and hold for three seconds if possible. Inhale, take a short break and repeat the process. If you are only able to complete one today, that's ok.

Continue to increase your quantity of crunches and the amount of time you tighten your abdomen muscles until you reach your goal. You may feel pain in your abdomen because you are working muscles that you don't usually work. As you continue, the pain should decrease. If a medical emergency arises while completing this exercise, discontinue and seek medical attention immediately.

Some of you have struggled with losing weight for a long time. You have tried programs that promised weight loss only to gain the weight back you lost. Managing your weight is a life time event. As with any program, _what you get out of a weight management program is based on what you put in it._ If you are serious about managing your weight, change your lifestyle and live a healthier life. I am wishing all of you success in achieving your _desired_ weight.

Contact Me

I hope my book was what you were looking for, and you can't wait to tell your friends about it. After you have participated in the program for a while, please post a review at www.Amazon.com.

Visit my website: https://www.stephenmwrightbooks.com

Like my Facebook page – www.facebook.com/stephenmwrightbooks

Email me - swright1068@gmail.com

References

1. Merriam-Webster Dictionary
   A: Definition of Overweight

2. Wikipedia, the free encyclopedia
   A: SMART criteria

THE GREATEST ACCOMPLISHMENTS STARTED WITH A SMALL DREAM

If you can dream it, you can achieve it. If your dream is to lose weight and keep it off, it doesn't matter if you have failed one hundred times. Never give up on your dream. Try, try, and try again, and one day, your dream will be fulfilled.

Printed in Great Britain
by Amazon

45027632R00020